Adel Bouguezzi

Potentially malignant oral lesions

Adel Bouguezzi

Potentially malignant oral lesions

ScienciaScripts

Imprint
Any brand names and product names mentioned in this book are subject to trademark, brand or patent protection and are trademarks or registered trademarks of their respective holders. The use of brand names, product names, common names, trade names, product descriptions etc. even without a particular marking in this work is in no way to be construed to mean that such names may be regarded as unrestricted in respect of trademark and brand protection legislation and could thus be used by anyone.

Cover image: www.ingimage.com

This book is a translation from the original published under ISBN 978-620-6-69358-1.

Publisher:
Sciencia Scripts
is a trademark of
Dodo Books Indian Ocean Ltd. and OmniScriptum S.R.L publishing group

120 High Road, East Finchley, London, N2 9ED, United Kingdom
Str. Armeneasca 28/1, office 1, Chisinau MD-2012, Republic of Moldova, Europe
Managing Directors: Ieva Konstantinova, Victoria Ursu
info@omniscriptum.com

Printed at: see last page
ISBN: 978-620-8-58029-2

Table of contents

Introduction

Potentially malignant conditions of the oral mucosa are also indicators of the risk of potential (clinically apparent) malignancies of the oral mucosa, and not just site-specific predictors.

The prognosis of potentially malignant lesions of the oral mucosa depends on their early detection and diagnosis.

Pre-cancerous conditions are the lesional consequences of certain diseases on the oral mucosa. The main pre-cancerous conditions are: certain clinical forms of lichen planus, bacterial (tertiary syphilis) and viral (HPV) infections, Plummer-Vinson syndrome (epithelial atrophy), and florid oral papillomatosis.

The normal oral mucosa consists of : - a multi-layered squamous epithelium with varying degrees of keratinization; - a basement membrane representing the interface between the epithelium and the chorion; - a chorion made up of loose connective tissue containing collagen fibers, elastic fibers, lymphocytes, plasmatocytes, vessels, nerves and accessory salivary glands.

Dysplasia, known as oral intraepithelial neoplasia (OIN), corresponds to a general alteration of the epithelium, with cells showing varying degrees of atypia, and involvement not extending beyond the basement membrane. OIN 1, or mild dysplasia, and OIN 2, moderate dysplasia, are defined as potentially reversible (removal of the causative agent) and with a malignancy potential $\leq$ 1%, and OIN 3, severe dysplasia, with an estimated malignancy potential of 11%.

Diagnosis of oral lesions is based on an accurate history and clinical examination, as well as further investigations. The toluidine blue test , cytological examination and biopsy are the most common. The now obsolete toluidine blue test looks for the presence of atypical, nucleic acid-rich cells that strongly absorb the dye. Cytological examination, or exfoliative cytology, is performed on a sample obtained by scraping epithelial cells spread out on a slide. This easy-to-perform technique is indicated for lesions such as candidiasis or bullous lesions, but not for precancerous lesions, due to the many false negatives. Only biopsy, which provides a histopathological study of the tissue removed for diagnostic purposes, remains the reference examination.

1. Histological approach to carcinogenesis

1·1· Histological overview of the oral mucosa

The oral mucosa is continuous with the cutaneous tissue of the face and lips. It lines the oral cavity and the inner surface of the lips, and continues posteriorly with the oropharyngeal mucosa. It surrounds the teeth, creating a watertight junction at the sulcus (epithelial attachment).The color of the mucosa is the result of a combination of factors: the thickness of the epithelium and the degree of keratinization make the mucosa whiter; the quantity of melanin is responsible for the physiological color of the mucosa; the concentration and dilation of small blood vessels in the underlying connective tissue, or atrophy of the epithelium, give the mucosa an erythematous appearance.

There are three types of oral mucosa depending on its topography:

* ***the masticatory mucosa***: covers the gums and hard palate. It plays a compressive role and supports mechanical loads during mastication. The epithelium is keratinized on the surface and contains long epithelial ridges that invaginate deep into the chorion, providing solid anchorage and preventing any mobility of the mucosa in relation to the deeper planes. There is no sub-mucosa.

****border covering mucosa***: covers most of the oral cavity, including the inner surface of the cheeks, the floor of the mouth, the ventral surface of the tongue, the soft palate and the labial mucosa. Its epithelium is not keratinized, and has faint epithelial ridges. The richly vascularized connective tissue is underpinned by a loose submucosa, giving it a degree of tissue flexibility.

* ***the specialized mucosa***: found on the tongue, it features various papillae: filiform and fungiform on the dorsal surface of the tongue, caliciform

forming the lingual v, and foliated papillae on the posterior lateral surfaces formed of lymphoid tissue.

The oral mucosa consists of a lining epithelium separated from the connective tissue (chorion) by a basement membrane.

- ✓ **Epithelial tissue:**

The epithelium of the oral mucosa is a stratified squamous squamous epithelium, keratinized in the masticatory mucosa and dorsal surface of the tongue, and non-keratinized in the bordering mucosa. The epithelium is made up of several layers of cells (keratinocytes) tightly bound together by desmosomes (spiny layer), ensuring strong cohesion between the cells.

Keratinocytes multiply in the basal layer, known as the germinal layer, where they are cubic in shape. They then progressively flatten out and migrate towards the superficial layers, replacing the cells eliminated by desquamation. During migration into the malpighian mucous body (spinous layer), the cells undergo maturation and differentiation, which determines whether the epithelium is keratinized or not.

There are two types of keratinization:

- **Orthokeratosis:** the flattened cells of the keratinized layer have lost their nuclei. They are preceded by a thin granular layer containing fine keratohyalin granules.
- **Parakeratosis:** stratum corneum cells retain a picnotic nucleus

- ✓ **The basal membrane :**

It separates the epithelium from the chorion, plays a fundamental role in epithelial-conjunctival exchanges and serves as an attachment for keratinocytes, which insert themselves into this membrane via hemidesmosomes.

✓**Connective tissue :**

The connective tissue or chorion supports the epithelium. It is composed of fibroblasts, immune cells, various fibers (collagen, elastic), blood vessels and nerve elements, contained within an amorphous fundamental substance.

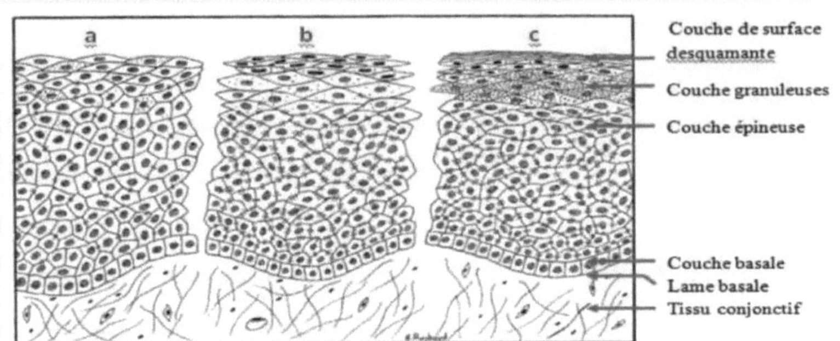

Figure 1: Epithelial composition as a function of keratinization

1·2· Natural history and biology of cancer

The word tumor (or neoplasm/neoplasia) characterizes a pathological tissue neoformation as distinct from an inflammatory process.

There are 2 types of neoplasm

* **Benign**: made up of cells identical to the initial tissue, which it displaces without destroying. It does not metastasize.

* **Malignant**: unlike a benign neoplasm, this is a tissue mass with metastatic potential that invades and destroys neighboring structures.

The proliferating cells may be identical to or different from the initial cells.

1·2·1· Cellular mechanisms of carcinogenesis

In carcinogenesis, a series of events transforms a physiological tissue into cancerous tissue, with the accumulation of genetic alterations and the acquisition of cancerous properties. The existence of genomic instability is a prerequisite for the alterations typical of cancer. Mutations are then promoted by the intervention of exogenous factors.

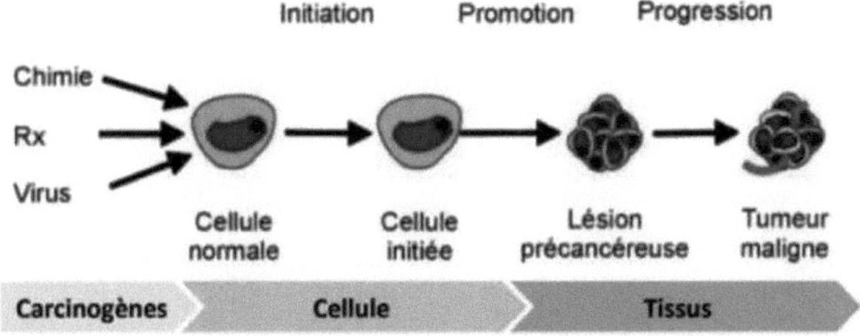

Source : Centre François Baclesse, Centre de lutte contre le cancer (Caen).

Figure 2: Illustration of carcinogenesis

1·2·2· Histological aspects

There are various stages of cellular and tissue alteration that can be identified upstream of the confirmed CE state. The latter may be preceded by a precancerous state: epithelial dysplasia or intraepithelial neoplasia (IEN).

They include :

* Disruption of physiological epithelial architecture ;

*Cytonuclear atypia, which may be criteria for malignancy;

* Mitotic activity qualitatively altered and quantitatively increased ;

* Faulty cell maturation, sometimes with dyskeratosis.

These anomalies can be prioritized according to several criteria:

- Epithelial height they occupy
- Importance of atypia
- Mitosis appearance

The 2005 World Health Organization (WHO) classification is the most widely used:

Table 1: WHO classification of epithelial dysplasia

	Description	Aspect histologique	Réversibilité
OIN 1 Dysplasie légère	▪ Cantonnée au tiers basal de la couche épithéliale ▪ Atypies cellulaires discrètes ▪ Mitoses normales		**Oui** Si suppression du/des agents causaux (tabac, alcool, etc.) + mesures d'hygiènes Si pas de régression, exérèse avec marge initiale de 1 à 3 mm
OIN 2 Dysplasie modérée	▪ Atteint jusqu'à 2/3 de la hauteur épithéliale ▪ Atypies cellulaires modérées ▪ Mitoses souvent normales, parfois anormales		
OIN 3 Dysplasie sévère - Carcinome In Situ (CIS)	▪ Hauteur épithéliale totale ▪ Atypies cellulaires marquées ▪ Mitoses très souvent anormales ▪ Anaplasie cellulaire (dédifférenciation) ▪ On parle à ce stade de **carcinome in situ** (CIS) ou **intraépithélial**	Source : Muller, « Oral epithelial dysplasia, atypical verrucous lesions and oral potentially malignant disorders : focus on histopathology », 2018.	**Non** Nécessité d'exérèse en bloc avec marges périphériques de 5 mm d'emblée, jusqu'au plan musculaire [33]

2. Risk factors

2.1. Tobacco

The strong association between cancers of the oral cavity and tobacco consumption is well established.

Tobacco also has an impact on the oral cavity, on saliva, periodontium and teeth, as well as on oral mucosa. It causes various mucosal lesions - benign, precancerous or cancerous.

Epidemiological studies show that the risk of developing oral cancer is five to nine times higher for smokers than for non-smokers, and this risk can increase up to 17 times for very heavy smokers of 80 cigarettes or more a day.

What's more, patients treated for oral cancer who continue to smoke are two to six times more likely to develop a second malignant tumour of the upper aerodigestive tract than those who stop smoking.

2·2· Alcohol

75% of people suffering from oral cancer are alcohol consumers. As with tobacco, the risk of developing this cancer is 6 times higher among drinkers. Alcohol is a risk factor for oral squamous cell carcinoma. It increases the permeability of the oral epithelium, acts as a solvent for tobacco carcinogens, induces basal cell proliferation and generates free radicals and acetaldehyde, which have the capacity to cause DNA damage.

Acetaldehyde is one of the primary metabolites of ethanol, and is the critical agent by which prolonged and excessive consumption of alcoholic beverages increases the risk of oral squamous cell carcinoma. Alcohol also acts synergistically with tobacco combustion products in the pathogenesis of oral squamous cell carcinoma.

2·3· Betel quid

In India and Southeast Asia, chronic use of betel quid (paan) in the mouth has been strongly associated with an increased risk of oral cancer. Betel quid generally consists of a betel leaf wrapped around a mixture of areca nuts and slaked lime, usually with tobacco and sometimes with sweeteners and condiments.

Hydrated lime causes the release of an alkaloid from the areca nut, which produces a feeling of euphoria and well-being in the user.

Betel quid chewing often leads to a progressive, scarring precancerous state of the mouth, known as oral submucosal fibrosis. In India, one study showed a 7.6% malignant transformation rate for oral submucosal fibrosis.

2.4 Age

Potentially malignant lesions are more frequent in older people (45 and over), due to their longer exposure to risk factors.

2.5 Oral hygiene

Poor oral hygiene contributes to the development of potentially malignant lesions.

2.6 Sun

Sun exposure increases the risk of potentially malignant lip lesions (chronic actinic cheilitis).

This is particularly true for people who work in the sun for long periods, such as farmers. People with pale complexions are also more likely to be affected. Most of these lip lesions appear on the lower lip, probably because this lip is more exposed to the sun.

2.7 Virus

Recent data suggest that human papillomavirus (HPV) may be associated with certain cancers of the mouth and oropharynx. HPV-16 has been detected in up to 22 percent of oral cancers, and HPV-18 has been detected in up to 14 percent of cases.

2.8 Weakened immune system

Patients with diminished immune defenses (e.g. under chronic immunosuppressive therapy or chemotherapy) are less able to defend themselves against the appearance, growth and spread of a potentially malignant lesion.

2·9· Disease) genetic

Certain diseases genetically predispose to an increased susceptibility to potentially malignant lesions of the oral cavity. This is the case for diseases characterized by high chromosomal fragility, such as Li Fraumeni syndrome or Xeroderma Pigmentosum.

3. Screening for potentially malignant lesions

Cancers of the oral cavity (lip, mouth without pharynx) are a public health priority. The Francim Registry recorded 7,500 new cases and 1,875 deaths in 2005 (INVS 2005 and 2000: lip, mouth and pharynx cancers). These cancers always have a poor prognosis: the five-year survival rate is around 40%. This rate has remained unchanged since 1989 (Francim network registries, 2007), due to insufficient early detection. Seventy percent of these cancers are diagnosed late at stage T3 or T4, resulting in mutilating and costly treatment. Diagnostic aids have improved detection (toluidine blue staining, chemiluminescence, fluorescence) or favored early detection of malignant transformation (transepithelial brushing, DNA tests, molecular markers).

Tissue **autofluorescence (FA)** is particularly suitable for identifying suspicious lesions in the oral mucosa. The technique is simple, non-invasive and inexpensive.

3·1· Le VELscope

The VELscope is a cutting-edge technology that is literally revolutionizing the way dentists detect oral cancer. It helps the dentist to make a precise and rapid diagnosis. It facilitates examination of the oral mucosa for abnormal lesions and precancerous cells.

3·1·1· The principle

The principle of FA visualization is based on the excitation of tissue fluorophores by a light beam of a given wavelength, and observation of the photon emission. Depending on the excitation wavelength, different fluorophores can be excited. Blue light with a wavelength between 400 and 460 nm will excite the tissue fluorophores of collagen and the redox cofactors of the flavin adenine dinucleotide/nicotinamide adenine dinucleotide phosphate (FAD/NADPH) system, which emit green light. Keratin and fibrin fluoresce light green, while bacterial porphirins fluoresce orange. In the case of tissue damage, the loss of fluorescence characterizes the destruction of collagen fibers and a decrease in FAD concentration due to increased tissue metabolic activity. However, loss of fluorescence can also correspond to the presence of hemoglobin or melanin. Many factors modify fluorescence, which raises questions about the sensitivity and specificity of this examination in the diagnosis of potentially malignant lesions and cancers of the oral cavity.

3·1·2· Procedure

1. It all starts with a visual examination of the oral cavity, lower face and neck;
2. The mouth is then cleaned with a rinse solution for one minute;
3. The patient is provided with protective eyewear, and the office lights are dimmed to give a better view of the oral cavity illuminated by the VELscope;
4. The dentist directs the device's blue light onto all the structures in the mouth;
5. If a lesion is detected, a biopsy can be taken on the spot for analysis.

3·1·3· VELscope benefits

- Quick and easy to use;
- Comfortable for the patient and completely pain-free;
- Safe;
- Can be combined with digital photography;
- Precise detection of precancerous and cancerous lesions invisible to

the naked eye.

4. Clinical forms of potentially malignant lesions

4·1· Terminology reminder

Lesions of the oral mucosa can take on different clinical forms, often in the form of several coexisting elementary lesions.

Table 2: elementary lesions of the oral mucosa

	Description	Taille
Macule	Tâche (blanche, rouge ou pigmentée) ± ronde, sans relief ni infiltration, dans le même plan que les tissus voisins.	< 1 cm
Plage, placard		> 1 cm
Papule	Lésion en relief, pleine, saillante, circonscrite, ± ronde, ferme à la palpation et de contenu non liquidien.	< 1 cm
Plaque		> 1 cm
Nodule	Élevure solide, ± circonscrite, ± saillante, ± ronde, de contenu non liquidien et profonde (du chorion). Souvent liée à une atteinte inflammatoire, réactionnelle ou tumorale.	
Végétation	Lésion faite d'excroissances, de morphologie variable, qui donne des aspects filiformes ou lobulés (en chou-fleur, en doigt de gant). Base sessile ou pédiculée. Peut s'ulcérer ou se kératiniser.	
Pustule	Lésion plane ou en relief, de couleur blanche à jaunâtre, contenant une sérosité de pus franc.	
Vésicule	Soulèvement épithélial translucide traduisant une micro-collection intra-épithéliale de liquide clair ou jaunâtre, laissant s'écouler une sérosité et évoluant en érosion après perçage de son toit.	< 0,2 cm
Bulle	Collection liquidienne contenant un liquide clair, jaunâtre ou hémorragique s'écoulant après perçage. Siège de la bulle soit intra- soit sous-épithélial. Toit fragile et transitoire évoluant en une érosion ou ulcération avec frange épidermique périphérique.	> 0,2 cm
Érosion	Perte de substance circonscrite et superficielle, intra-épithéliale, décrivant une lésion en creux à bords ± réguliers, à fond érythémateux et guérissant sans séquelle cicatricielle.	
Ulcération	Perte de substance ± profonde avec destruction de l'épithélium et du conjonctif, à fond fibrineux.	

Source : Kuffer et al., *La muqueuse buccale de la clinique au traitement*, 2009.

4·2· Let potentially malignant lesions

4·2·1· Leukoplakia [1,14]

Oral leukoplakias are considered to be the most common potentially malignant diseases of the oral cavity.

They define white, non-detachable lesions that can appear on all mucous membranes (keratinized or non-keratinized) and are not associated with a known disease or trauma.

o ***Diagnosis***

The diagnosis of oral leukoplakia is clinical, and is made after all other diagnostic hypotheses for white lesions have been ruled out. It is a diagnosis of elimination.

There are two types: **homogeneous** and **inhomogeneous:**

Distinction is based on color and surface morphology (thickness and texture).

***homogenous** :

A white lesion is said to be homogeneous if there is no variation in color and/or thickness.

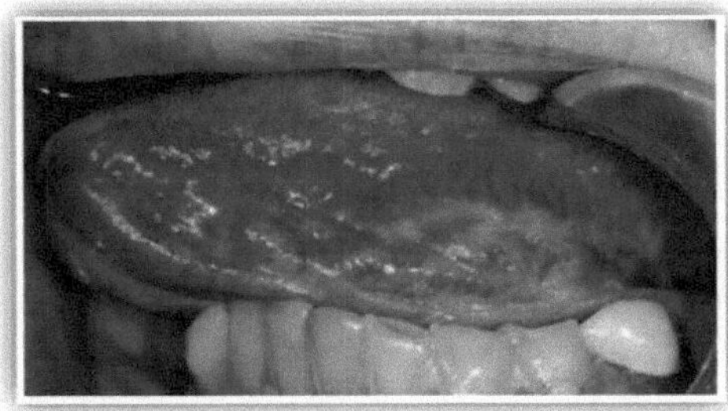

Figure 3: An area of homogeneous leukoplakia with a flat, thin surface and uniformly white appearance affecting the ventrolateral tongue region. The color and appearance mimic white paint brushed over the mucosa.

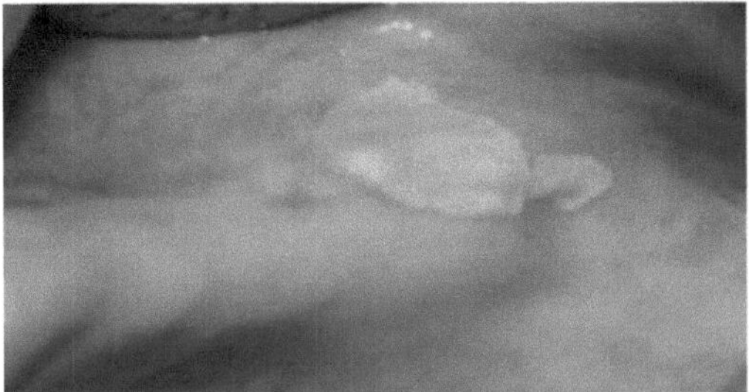

Figure 4: Idiopathic homogeneous leukoplakia (non-smoking patient). White plaque on the alveolar mucosa overhanging the edentulous ridge, posterior left sector. The removable full denture fits perfectly.

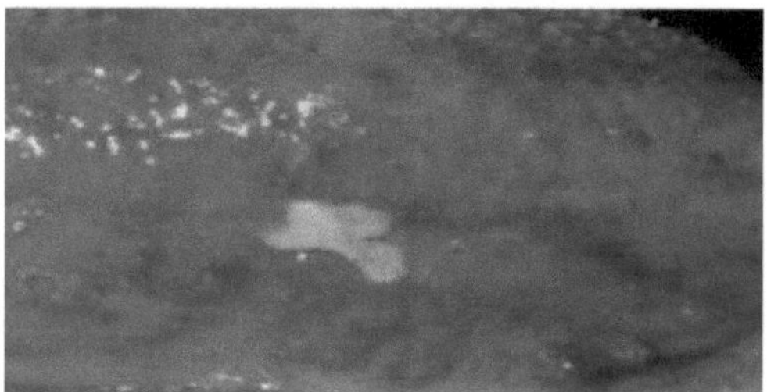

Figure 5: Homogeneous leukoplakia caused by smoking.

***Inhomogeneous**: a white lesion is said to be inhomogeneous if it presents areas of differing thickness, or if the white part is associated with erythema, erosion or ulceration. Erosion is superficial loss of substance without destruction of the underlying chorion. An ulceration is a deep loss of substance involving all or part of the chorion.

Non-homogeneous varieties include **3 clinical types** and are generally symptomatic:

1. **Speckled** - mixed, white and red (also called erythroleukoplakia), but predominantly white.
2. **Nodular**: small, polypoid, rounded, red or white excrescences.

3. **Verrucous or exophytic** - wrinkled or wavy surface.

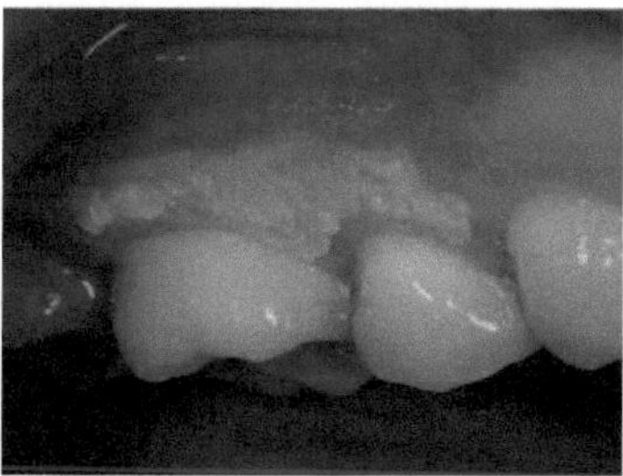

Figure 6: A small area of verrucous leukoplakia on the attached gingiva. Note the wavy, verrucous appearance of the lesion.

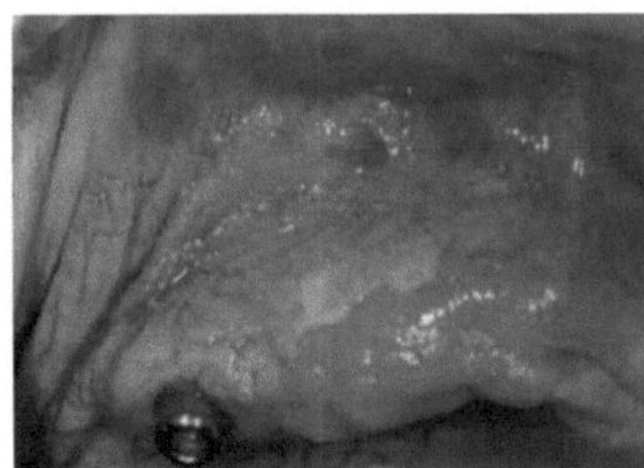

Figure 7: Proliferative verrucous leukoplakia affecting gingiva, alveolar and buccal mucosa

NB: Inhomogeneous Ieukoplakia has a poorer prognosis than homogeneous Ieukoplakia, as it carries a higher risk of malignant transformation.

o ***Histology***

The histological appearance is comparable whatever the origin of the Ieukoplakia (smoking or idiopathic), and does not distinguish an Ieukoplakia from a white lesion of traumatic origin. The white color corresponds to hyperkeratosis (increase in the ortho- or para-keratinized epithelial layer for physiologically keratinized mucosa such as the palate, gingiva and dorsal surface of the tongue; appearance of an ortho- or para-keratinized epithelial layer for physiologically non-keratinized mucosa such as the cheeks, ventral surface of the tongue and floor of the mouth).

o ***Evolution***

The evolution of oral leukoplakia is not predictable, and depends on many individual factors. However, some broad trends can be identified. Idiopathic leukoplakia may regress for no apparent reason. It may also spread or change, as is the case with most leukoplakias of smoking origin (outside the context of smoking cessation). The risk of transformation into carcinoma is not negligible. The incidence of malignant transformation of leukoplakia lesions ranges from 0.1% to 17%, depending on the study. Smoking combined with alcoholism significantly increases the likelihood of carcinoma.

Thus, the appearance of pain, adenopathy, induration, or a change in the texture, appearance, relief or extent of the initial white lesion should raise fears of a cancerous transformation, and necessitate a biopsy to look for dysplasia at best, or carcinoma at worst.

However, it is important to note that dysplasia is not a necessary condition for malignant transformation, which can occur in the absence of dysplasia. Similarly, a carcinoma may appear on homogeneous leukoplakia or healthy mucosa without intermediate tissue changes.

Table3: showing the degrees of dysplasia (cell differentiation disorder). The degree of dysplasia is determined by the height of the affected epithelial zone, the extent of cellular atypia and the appearance of mitosis.

Dysplasie légère	Trouble ne dépassant pas le tiers de la hauteur de l'épithélium. Atypies cellulaires discrètes, mitoses normales.
Dysplasie modérée	Trouble intéressant plus du tiers et jusqu'à 70 % de la hauteur de l'épithélium. Atypies cellulaires modérées, mitoses normales ou anormales.
Dysplasie sévère Carcinome *in situ*	Trouble > à 70 % de la hauteur de l'épithélium. Atypies cellulaires marquées, mitoses souvent anormales. Le terme carcinome *in situ* est employé quand toute la hauteur de l'épithélium est atteinte mais en présence d'une membrane basale encore intacte.

4·2·2·trythroplαsie (4,19,14)

Erythroplasia of the oral mucosa is still considered the lesion with the highest potential for malignant transformation.

Some authors no longer consider it a potentially malignant lesion, since cancer is already present in the vast majority of cases.

o ***Clinical manifestation :***

- Appears as a bright red macule or patch with a velvety texture.
- Typically soft to palpation, with induration only observed in cases of malignancy.
- Lesions usually have an irregular but well-defined outline. Occasionally, however, the surface may appear granular.
- There are usually no symptoms. Patients may report non-specific pain or burning of the area. A metallic taste sensation has also been reported.
- The floor of the mouth, ventral surface of the tongue, soft palate, tonsils and buccal mucosa are the most frequently affected sites.
- Lesions are generally small (less than 1.5 cm), but larger lesions have been reported (>4 cm).
- Erythroplasia rarely affects several sites.
- In the event of malignant transformation, patients may present signs and symptoms of oral squamous cell carcinoma (OSCC).

- There is no recognized classification of erythroplasia.

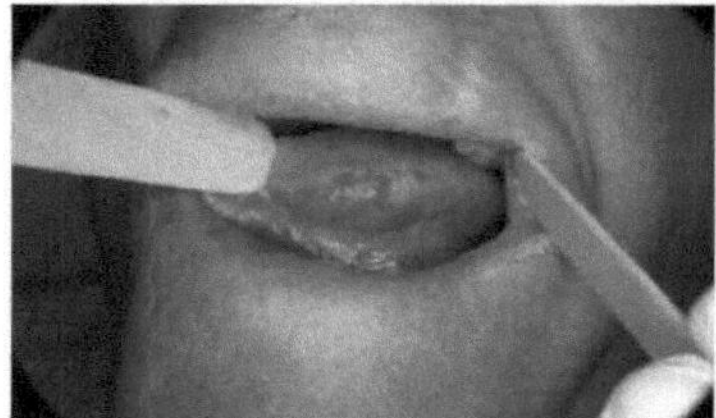
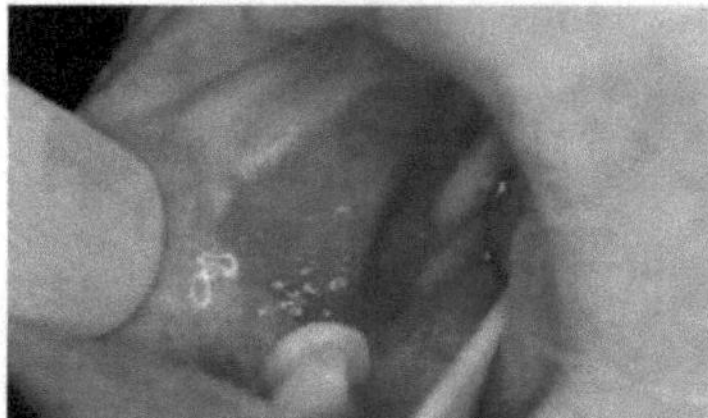

Figure 8: Generalized erythroplasia homogeneously affecting the left lateral border of the tongue and homogeneous erythroplasia affecting the posterior right buccal mucosa (19).

o ***<u>Diagnosis</u>***

- An isolated lesion with well-defined margins helps the practitioner to distinguish erythroplasia clinically from other conditions.
- These isolated lesions may be discovered incidentally by dentists, prompting referral.
- A biopsy must be performed as a matter of urgency and is essential to exclude neoplastic transformation.
- The histopathological features that can be found have been described above: thin, atrophied epithelium, absence of keratin and hyperplasia. Hematoxylin and eosin are the stains most commonly used by histopathologists to diagnose erythroplasia.

o ***<u>Malignant transformation:</u>***

- The rate of malignant transformation varies from 14 to 50%.
- Many red lesions may present with carcinoma in situ or invasive carcinoma at the time of diagnosis.
- The presence of moderate to severe dysplasia indicates a considerably higher risk of malignant transformation.
- A recent systematic review reported that the overall risk of malignant transformation was 33.1%, and the rate of malignant transformation

per year was 2.7%.

o ***Histology :***

*Maximum epithelial atrophy at the roof of the chorion papillae, with no surface keratinization.

*Chorionic abnormalities.

*Epithelial dysplasia lesions characterized by the presence of large cells with vesicular, nucleolated nuclei and clear, sometimes dyskeratotic cytoplasm.

4·2·3· Palatal lesions of inverted smokers [4]

This condition is specific to people who smoke with the glowing end of the cigarette in their mouth.

Lesions are palatal, red, white or mixed.

There is no difficulty in defining or diagnosing these lesions once the habit has been identified in an individual or a community.

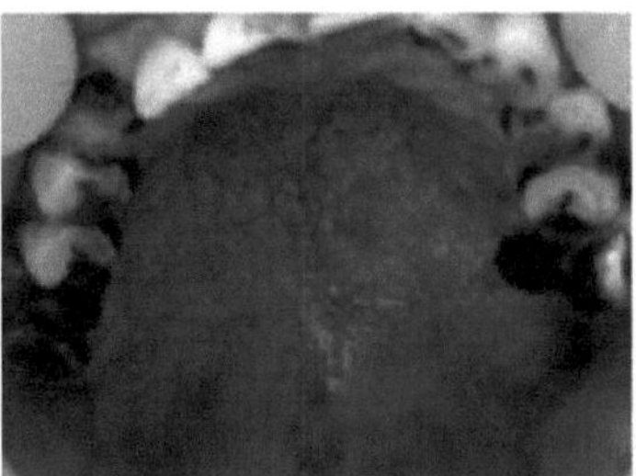

Figure 9: Severe palate changes associated with upside-down smoking habit

4·2·4· Submucosal fibrosis [",,s,4,19]

Submucosal fibrosis is a chronic disease of the oral cavity, mainly observed in India, but also in other parts of Asia.

It is thought to be linked to spicy eating habits, B vitamin deficiencies, betel nut chewing and smoking.

The disease is most common between the ages of 20 and 40. The rate of malignant transformation is around 0.5-6%.

o ***Clinical manifestation***

Clinically, submucosal fibrosis results in an intense burning sensation and the formation of vesicles (especially on the palate and tongue) followed by superficial ulcerations.

The fibrous stage is characterized by a whitening of the mucosa, which appears smooth, atrophies and gradually loses its elasticity.

Mobility is limited and areas of papillary atrophy are observed, sometimes in the vicinity of keratotic plaques.

The palate, tonsil cavity and entire oral mucosa may be affected, as well as the pharynx and esophagus.

Opening the mouth, chewing and swallowing become difficult.

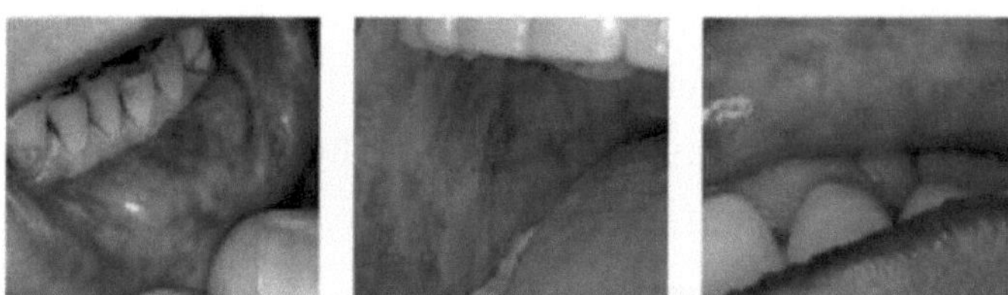

Figure 10: Fibrosis of the oral mucosa

4.2.5. Actinic cheilites [(4)]

Actinic cheilitis is a lip disorder considered potentially malignant. The vermilion epithelium may be hyperplastic or atrophic, with maturation abnormalities, varying degrees of keratinization, cellular atypia and high mitotic activity. The underlying connective tissue shows basophilic collagen degeneration and elastosis.

Presumptive clinical diagnosis must be confirmed by biopsy.

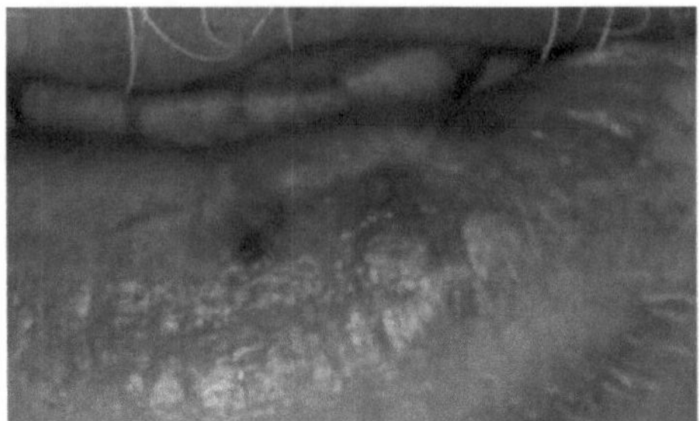

Figure 11: Scab on the lower labial half-mucosa, present for 6 months. Note the reworked appearance of the entire half-mucosa, suggesting actinic cheilitis.

4.2.6. Lichen planus [4,17,18]

Lichen planus (LP) is a benign, chronic inflammatory skin and mucous membrane disease, most likely due to an autoimmune mechanism. It is not an infectious disease.

The initial clinical description by Wilson in 1869 and the histological description by Dubreuil in 1906 is characterized by a keratinization disorder, with polymorphous clinical aspects.

o **Clinical manifestation**

In the oral cavity, the disease takes on a clinical appearance somewhat different from that of the skin, and is characterized by lesions consisting of white, gray, velvety, filiform radiating papules, arranged linearly, annular and retiforme, forming typical lacy and reticular plaques.

A small, raised white dot is present at the intersection of the white lines known here as Wickham striae, compared with the Wickham striae in the skin.

Lesions are asymptomatic, occurring bilaterally/symmetrically throughout the oral cavity, but are more common on the buccal mucosa, tongue, lips, gums, floor of the mouth and palate, and may appear weeks or months before the onset of skin lesions. There are six clinical forms:

1- ***Reticular: This is*** the most common clinical form of the disease, and presents as a fine, asymptomatic, intertwined lace-like pattern called "Wickham's striae" in a bilaterally symmetrical form, involving the posterior mucosa of the cheek in most cases.

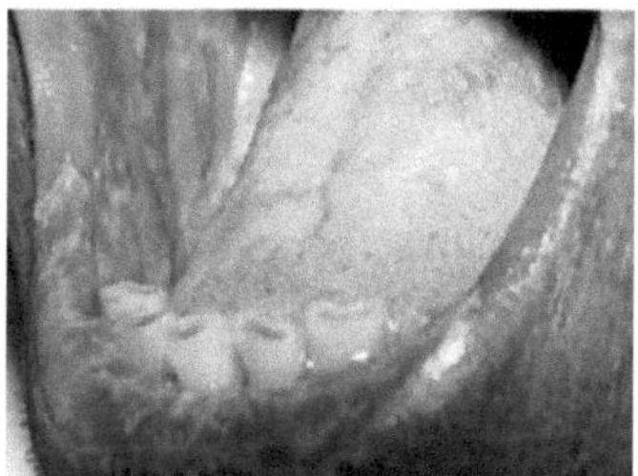

Figure 12: Reticular shape

2- ***Erosive:*** This is the most important form of the disease, presenting symptomatic lesions often surrounded by fine, radiating keratinized streaks with a reticular appearance.

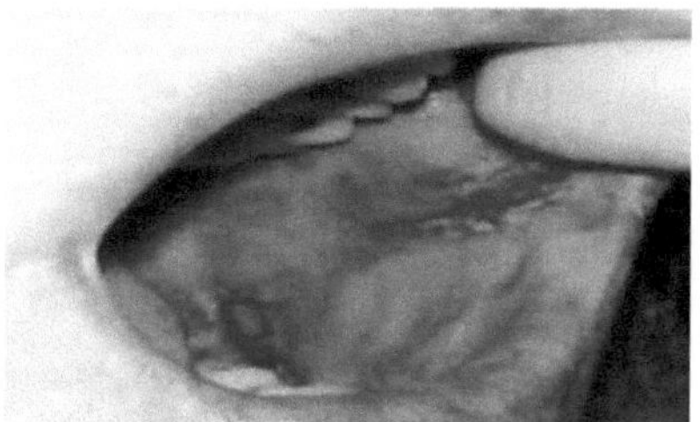

Figure 13: Erosive form

3- ***Atrophic:*** It presents diffuse red lesions and may resemble the combination of two clinical forms, such as the presence of white striae characteristic of the reticular type surrounded by an erythematous zone.

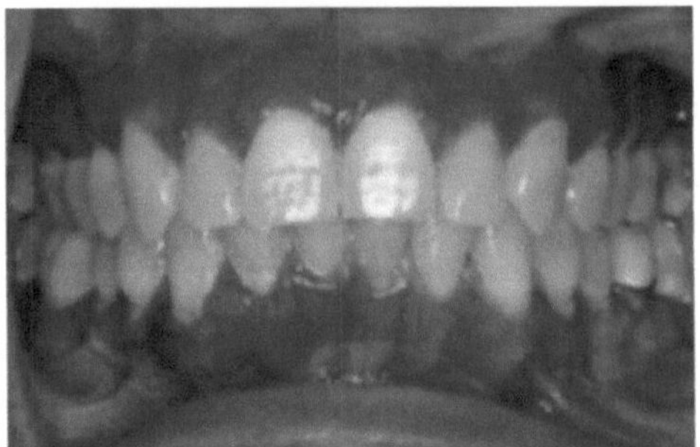

Figure 14: Atrophic form

4- ***Plaque-like:*** This type presents homogeneous, whitish irregularities similar to leukoplakia, mainly on the back of the tongue and cheek mucosa.

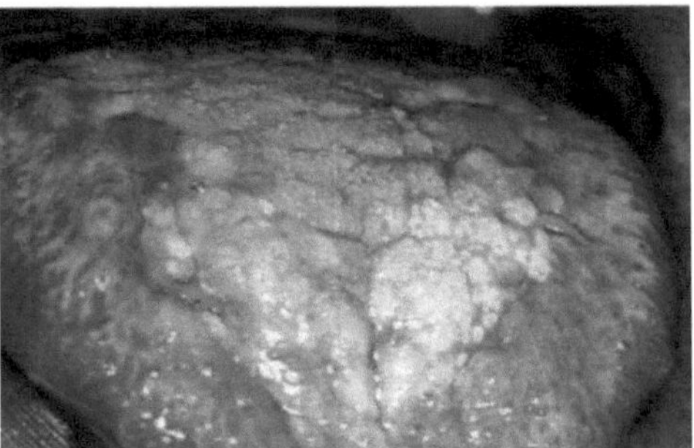

Figure 15: Plate shape

5- ***Papular:*** This form is rarely observed and is normally followed by another type of variant described. It presents small white papules with fine striations at the periphery.

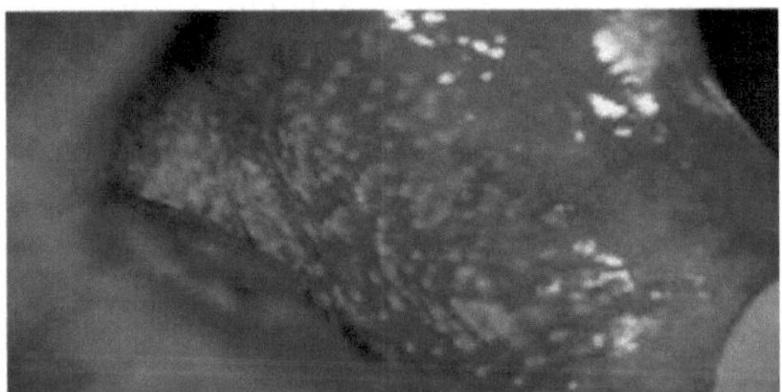

Figure 16: Papillary form

6- ***Bullous*:** This is the most unusual clinical form, presenting blisters that increase in size and tend to rupture, leaving the surface ulcerated and painful. Nikolsky's sign may be positive.

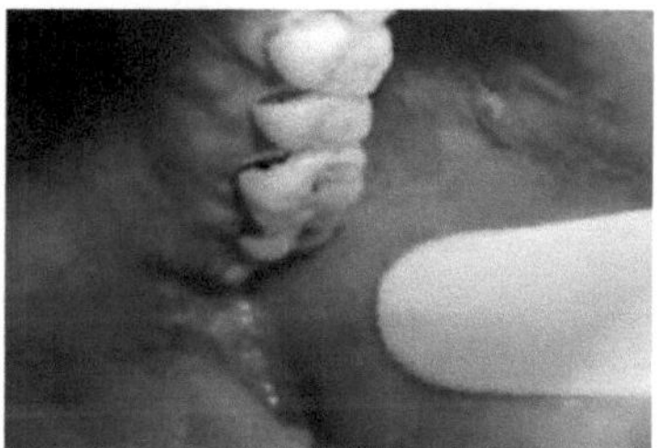

Figure 17: Bullous form

4·2·7· Discoid lupus erythematosus [4,18]

Discoid lupus erythematosus is a chronic autoimmune disorder of unknown etiology. The clinical distinction between discoid lupus erythematosus, lichen planus and erythroplasia is sometimes difficult. There is conflicting evidence as to whether this disease is potentially malignant. Cases of malignant transformation have been reported, most often in labial localization.

o **Clinical manifestation**

Oral lesions are present in around 20% of cases, generally affecting the lips, hard palate and buccal mucosa.

They are characterized by the presence of a central erythema or ulceration surrounded by hyperkeratotic papules or radiating striae, and peripheral telangiectasias. The "honeycomb" appearance appears in lesions of long duration.

Mucosal lesions may occur without skin involvement or before the development of skin lesions. Lesions on the lips may extend to the adjacent skin, obscuring the vermilion border.

desquamative gingivitis affecting the lower and/or upper gums may also be present.

With healing, erosive lesions may leave a post-inflammatory pigmentation.

The most common symptoms of SLE are burning, photosensitivity, dryness, sensitivity and pain, but lesions can be asymptomatic.

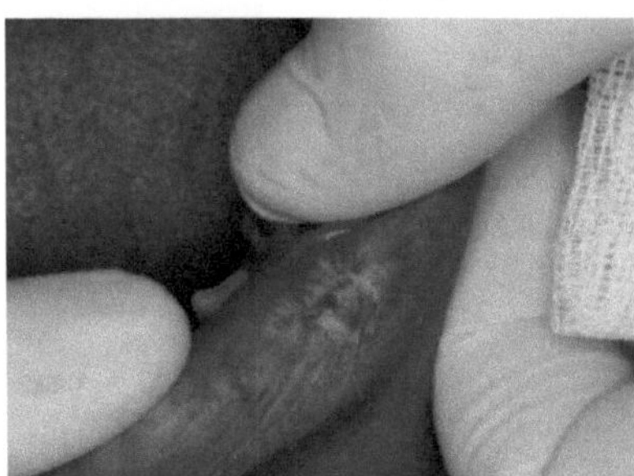

Figure 18:

4·2·8· Hereditary conditions [4]

Two conditions that can lead to an increased risk of cancer in the oral cavity are **dyskeratosis congenita** and **epidermolysis bullosa.** These are very rare hereditary diseases.

In X-linked dyskeratosis congenita, which only affects males, white patches on the dorsal surface of the tongue may be present. They are distinguished from leukoplakia by the absence of risk factors and the young age of patients, which points to a hereditary condition.

■ Congenital dyskeratosis

Characterized by more or less reticulated and atrophic keratotic and leuko-melano dermal skin lesions, nail dystrophy, early oral leukoplakia and severe hematological disorders.

■ Epidermolysis bullosa

Refers to a group of mostly hereditary diseases that lead to the formation of bullae and ulcerations on the skin and sometimes on the oral mucosa.

In almost all patients, lesions appear at birth or in early childhood, and there is often a family history.

Skin lesions are constantly present.

Some forms of epidermolysis bullosa can cause scarring and limit the opening of the mouth.

The diagnosis can be suspected quickly after birth, given the skin involvement and other possible manifestations.

Oral cavity biopsy and diagnostic aids :

Biopsy has become the standard method for diagnosing many lesions and conditions, including oral cancer and potentially malignant diseases [1]. Biopsy is defined as the removal of a fragment of tissue from a living organism for microscopic examination. It can be used to confirm a provisional diagnosis, to establish a definitive diagnosis, or to exclude differential diagnoses. In addition to diagnostic purposes, biopsy can be used to determine the efficacy of a treatment, or to establish a prognosis for malignant or premalignant lesions. Finally, the biopsy and histopathological report are legally valid documents [2, 3]. 2.2 Indications and contraindications for oral biopsy Indications for oral biopsy are based on a number of factors, including the clinical and macroscopic characteristics of the lesion, such as its evolution, macroscopic presentation and response to various treatments. It is always recommended in cases of suspected cancer. Table 1.2 details the indications and clinical presentations that require biopsy [4-6]. Contraindications are generally related to the patient's general state of health. Biopsy is not indicated for anatomical variants (e.g. lingual varicose vein, racial pigmentation, marginal exfoliative glossitis, linea alba, teeth marks on the tongue or Fordyce grains), irritant/traumatic lesions despite removal of the local irritant agent, and inflammatory or infectious lesions consequent upon specific local treatment [4, 6].

In some cases, it may be advisable to perform a biopsy on a lesion that is causing great concern in a patient, even if it does not appear suspicious to the healthcare professional. This is because you need to take the patient's expectations into account, and bear in mind that it "can't hurt" and may enable you to offer the patient the best treatment options. 2.3. Classification and types of oral cavity biopsy Biopsies can be classified into different sub-categories [2, 3]. Depending on the amount of tissue removed, they may be incisional (only a representative part of the lesion is removed) or excisional (the entire lesion is removed). Depending on the anatomical location of the lesion, biopsy may be direct (sampling from a superficial, easily accessible area) or indirect (if the lesion is deeper and covered by a layer of apparently healthy mucosa, which may require creating an access patch before the lesion can be sampled). Other categories are based, for example, on the specific instruments or techniques used (scalpel, punch, hollow needle), the treatment of the tissue removed (e.g. fresh, frozen, formalin-fixed and paraffin-embedded), the type of tissue removed (soft tissue, bone tissue, blood). In the following sections of this chapter, we will focus on the most common biopsies performed to diagnose OPMD [2, 3]. Soft-tissue biopsies For a soft-tissue biopsy, tissue is usually removed using a scalpel, punch or forceps, but lasers or an electric scalpel may also be used [2]. If the biopsy is performed for diagnostic purposes, a conventional scalpel or punch is preferable to lasers (diodes, Nd:YAG or CO2) or an electric scalpel, as the latter may alter the tissue, making diagnosis more difficult [7-10]. The Er:YAG laser is the most effective in terms of tissue preservation [7, 11]. Lasers are preferred for vascular abnormalities or patients with bleeding disorders, as they have a coagulant effect [11]. Care must always be taken to select the instrument that will be of most benefit to the patient, keeping in mind the objective, which is to remove tissue that can be used for biopsy. In most cases of OPMD, an incisional, excisional or punch biopsy is usually performed. 2.3.1. Incisional biopsy Incisional biopsy involves removing a representative part of the lesion (see Table 2.2). Ideally, the sample should contain a representative area of the lesion and adjacent tissues. Whether it is necessary to remove more healthy or abnormal tissue depends primarily on the nature of the lesion (e.g. in the case of suspected cancer, it is better to remove more abnormal tissue; in the case of a condition with swelling, it is preferable to remove more healthy adjacent tissue) [2, 4, 12, 13]. In the case of extensive or large lesions (length greater than approx. 1-2 cm) or multiple lesions, incisional or mapped biopsy may be indicated. In the case of heterogeneous lesions (in terms of color, texture or consistency), multiple incisional biopsies may be chosen to obtain different representations of the lesion. In this case, each sample must be identified and placed in a separate, identified container. Incisional biopsy is the best method for suspected cancer and potentially malignant oral lesions [2, 3, 14]. For biopsies of vascular lesions, close to neurovascular tissue (with a high risk of bleeding or numbness) or where access is difficult, it may be preferable to perform them in a hospital setting. An incisional biopsy should suffice for histopathological evaluation, and reduces the risk of tissue damage [2-4, 13]. To begin with, a full medical history of the disease should be taken, and the interior of the oral cavity thoroughly examined. This will help determine the most suspicious part of the lesion (spotted, red, hardened or warty): this is the part that should be removed for biopsy. It may be advisable to use diagnostic aids to identify the most representative part of the lesion to be biopsied (as described below) [2-4]. It is also essential to obtain the patient's informed consent, explaining the risks and benefits of biopsy. You should choose suitable instruments to minimize the risk of tissue damage, and administer an analgesic to the patient, at less than half a centimetre from the site of the lesion, to preserve the tissue. Don't hesitate to use retractors to clear the surgical field.

Using a scalpel (usually no. 15), make two incisions at 45° to the epithelial surface, converging towards each other to form an ellipse with two V-shaped ends. The length-to-width ratio should be approximately 3:1 to facilitate closure and promote good, scar-free healing. The axis of the ellipse's length should be parallel to the normal stretching direction of the mucosa, so that the incision is subjected to less tension, thus avoiding possible wound dehiscence. In addition, the incision should never be perpendicular to structures such as neurovascular bundles, to prevent the risk of damaging them. Avoid incising over necrotic tissue or the central part of an ulcer. You can use Adson forceps or sutures to remove tissue. 18 You can also use the suture to guide the removal [2-4]. Non-absorbable sutures are generally not indicated in the oral cavity. The sample should then be placed in a container marked with the patient's identification and filled with a fixation solution (formalin 10%), the volume of which should not exceed 10 to 20 times that of the sample. You must then attach a pathology requisition to the container and send it to the appropriate laboratory. Samples intended for immunofluorescence studies should not be fixed, but immersed in Michel's fixative or sent fresh, in a container itself transported in a freezer bag. Fresh tissue samples should be sent to the laboratory as soon as possible [24].

The request for pathological analysis must contain information on the lesion and the patient's medical history, including a brief history of the lesion, its clinical characteristics, risk factors (tobacco, alcohol, betel nut) and a predictive diagnosis, as well as the desired orientation for sampling and the type of biopsy performed (incisional or excisional). 2.3.2. Excisional biopsy An excisional biopsy involves removing the entire lesion, with a margin of adjacent healthy deeper tissue (Figure 2.2). In addition to small OPMDs, it is indicated for small lesions (approx. 1 cm), such as papillomas, fibromas, granulomas, or for vascular or focally pigmented lesions. Excisional biopsy not only enables histological analysis, but can also be used for treatment, as the entire lesion is removed [2-4]. Technically, excisional biopsy is very similar to incisional biopsy in terms of anesthesia, instruments used and incision. The difference is that particular attention must be paid to the margins. The incision must be made over healthy tissue, both lengthwise and in depth, and the margin must be clean. If the lesion is malignant, the margin must be larger. In the case of papilloma lesions, care must be taken to remove the base to avoid recurrence. Make sure you palpate the lesion to determine its depth [2-4]. If you suspect the presence of cancer, you can direct the sampling. 2.3.3. Biopsy with biopsy forceps or punch These instruments have been designed to facilitate sampling of superficial lesions. Biopsy forceps resemble tweezers with a sharp (bird's beak-shaped) tip, enabling incisional biopsy of a superficial lesion, without the need to close with sutures. It's ideal for hard-to-reach sites. The punch is equipped with an active cutting part similar to a circular scalpel. It is a single-use instrument, available in different diameters (2 to 10 mm). OPMD generally uses 4 to 6 mm punches. It is most often used for incisional biopsies, but for less extensive lesions, it can be used to perform an excisional biopsy. The technique for performing a punch biopsy is similar to that for incisional biopsies, described above (Table 2), but with a punch, the incision is made over the most representative part of the lesion, by applying gentle pressure and rotating the blade, along an axis perpendicular to the extent of the mucosa (Figure 2.3). The incised tissue may be extracted inside the punch cylinder itself, but generally speaking, you'll need to cut away the base of the tissue to be analyzed. In most cases, wound healing will be of the secondary type, which means you won't need to suture; however, if homeostasis proves difficult, you may settle for a stitch This type of biopsy is easy to perform for single or multiple biopsies of representative samples. The size of the sample to be analyzed depends on the size of the punch chosen. This technique is not recommended for more extensive lesions, lesions located near vascularized or nervous areas, or sites that are difficult to access, such as the hard palate.

2.4. Diagnostic aids Diagnostic aids are materials and/or devices that facilitate detection of the most abnormal part of an oral lesion to help the practitioner define where to perform the biopsy [1618]. They are generally non-invasive and can also be used to determine surgical margins in the case of excisional biopsy, or to monitor high-risk patients. In primary care, diagnostic tools can be used to detect any abnormal oral lesion, which can then be used as a reference to establish a definitive diagnosis of OPMD or oral cancer. In the context of secondary or tertiary care, they can help to better characterize and even map the disease of a patient suffering from OPMD, which is particularly useful in the case of extensive, multiple or heterogeneous lesions. This facilitates biopsy site selection at the start of treatment and during surveillance, and reduces the risk of a positive margin following excision of an OSCC or dysplastic lesion [16]. There are several types of diagnostic aid, including vital stain, optical or light-based systems, cytology or salivary tests. These are described in the sections below. We will also look at vibrational spectroscopy, a promising new diagnostic aid. 2.4.1. Vital dyes Vital dyes are biocompatible dyes used in a form similar to mouthwash, or as a topical, applied directly to the chosen site on the oral mucosa. They can be used to gather information on the various characteristics of a lesion, to identify an inconspicuous lesion and to select the most suitable site for a biopsy. In oral surgery, toluidine blue is most commonly used, but other dyes are described below [4, 15, 16]. Toluidine blue Toluidine blue (TB), also known as trimethylthionine hydrochloride, is a vital dye that has been used in oral surgery for over fifty years. TB is a cationic, metachromatic dye with a strong affinity for tissue acids such as nucleic acids. Areas where the mucosa shows abnormalities or dysplastic or anaplastic cells may retain more dye, making them darker blue (Figure 2.4). This can help detect satellite lesions, or lesions invisible to the naked eye [16, 18-20]. Toluidine blue is useful for selecting the area to be biopsied and determining the margins of the lesion (in the case of excision), and in the management of patients with a history of OSCC or OPMD [15, 16]. It is used as a 1% or 2% solution, or in ready-to-use packs. It is used in combination with a 1% acetic acid solution to remove any excess that does not cling to the tissue [15, 16, 19].

A recent meta-analysis revealed that toluidine blue, used as a single dye, had a sensitivity of 87% (95% CI: 80-94%) and a specificity of 71% (95% CI: 61-0.82%) [21]. False positives (inflamed tissue, ulcers) and false negatives can occur when the epithelium is thick and the dye fails to infiltrate, as in the case of hyperkeratotic lesions [16]. TB can be used to facilitate conventional oral auscultation, or preferably to complete a diagnosis. Methylene blue Methylene blue (MB), also known as methylthioninium chloride, is an aromatic heterocycle similar to TB. Like TB, it has affinities with acidic components, which facilitates its retention by dysplastic cells [16, 22, 23]. MB is used to detect possible cancerous lesions, notably in the prostate, bladder and gastrointestinal tract. It can also be used as a topical antiseptic agent in the treatment of certain diseases. In oral surgery, it is frequently used for staining purposes prior to endoscopy. It is also used in certain types of photodynamic therapy [16, 22-25]. The indications and methods of application are similar to those of TB, the difference being that MB may be more economical and less toxic [17, 18]. However, this dye has yet to really prove itself in the detection of oral cancers, so we need to do more studies on the subject. Lugol's solution Lugol's solution (LI), also known simply as ludol, or iodized water, is used as a reagent for the glycogen present in the cytoplasm of non-keratinized cells, giving it an orange-brown color. Thus, in the case of OPMD, if LI is applied to the lesion, the adjacent healthy mucosa turns brown, while the abnormal tissues do not turn brown at all. It can be used in combination with TB to stain abnormal tissue dark blue and healthy tissue brown. However, there are no serious studies to support the efficacy of LI in the diagnosis of OPMD [16, 26]. 22 Rose Bengal Rose Bengal (RB) is a fluorescein derivative. Used as a xanthene dye, it has photosensitive properties. It is mainly used to detect corneal damage, but could also be used with light as part of photodynamic therapy, or with sound technology as part of ultrasound treatment [16, 27, 28]. RB stains dead or degenerated cells, or even dysplastic or malignant cells, without staining healthy epithelial cells, thus revealing corneal lesions and conjunctival neoplastic lesions. There are very few data on the efficacy of this dye in the diagnosis of OPMD [16, 27, 28].

5. Care and maintenance

5·1· Preventive care

Risk factor modification, assessment and attempts to modify risk factor behavior are an integral part of any management protocol for potentially malignant conditions.

❖ **Smoking cessation** :

Although smoking is often considered the main risk factor. However, educational programs encouraging smoking cessation can lead to a decrease in the incidence of leukoplakia, and smoking cessation can result in the resolution of a fair number of leukoplakias.

❖ **Alcohol advice :**

Whether alcohol alone increases precancerous transformation is controversial, but there is clear evidence that alcohol availability and consumption are on the rise in most populations around the world.

Nevertheless, identifying patients with excessive alcohol consumption offers important educational and healthcare opportunities, and should be encouraged in all potentially malignant cases.

5·2· Curative care

5·2·1· Medical treatment

Some studies have reported a regression of leukoplakia after the use of vitamin A, local and systemic retinoids, and systemic beta-carotene.

5·2·2· Cryotherapy

This is a specialized technique involving the localized destruction of diseased tissue through the surgical application of extreme cold, usually liquid nitrogen.

5·2·3· Surgical excision and reconstruction

Surgical excision is the most commonly used treatment for potentially malignant lesions of the oral mucosa. Excision must be performed with a cold-blade scalpel, so that the lesion borders are not burned and can be analyzed by the anatomopathologist.

If dysplasia (moderate or severe) or cellular infiltration of the chorion is present, the patient should be referred to a hospital stomatology or maxillofacial surgery department. In these histological situations, surgical removal of the leukoplakia, anatomopathological analysis of the entire sample and long-term monitoring (there is a risk of recurrence) are indicated.

5·2·4· Interventional laser surgery

The CO2, Nd-YAG and KTP lasers have been used in conjunction with various vaporization or excision techniques for the treatment of oral leukoplakia, but recent years have seen the emergence of new lasers whose scope of application extends to other pathologies, including potentially malignant lesions of the oral mucosa.

Conclusion

The terms "precancerous", "precursor lesions", "pre-malignant", "intraepithelial neoplasia" and "potentially malignant pathologies" have been used in the international literature to describe tissue alterations within which cancer appears more frequently than in homologous normal tissue. Potentially malignant conditions of the oral mucosa are also indicators of the risk of potential (clinically apparent) malignancies of the oral mucosa, and not just site-specific predictors.

The dental surgeon must be attentive to the presence and evolution of these lesions. His medical and legal responsibility is fully engaged.

The prognosis of potentially malignant lesions of the oral mucosa depends on their early detection and diagnosis. Their detection is usually based on a valuable clinical examination, supplemented by anatomopathological examination.

References

1- Dr Nathan MOREAU, Emilie VAUCARD, Dr Anne-Laure Ejeil

Oral leukoplakia: potentially malignant lesions

LE FIL DENTAIRE; N°73, May 2012

2- practical tips for encology

Benign, precancerous and cancerous lesions of the oral cavity

JSOP / n° 4 / April 2011

3- https://www.sciencedirect.com/science/article/abs/pii/S0035176810001968

4- L Ben Slama.

Potentially malignant conditions of the oral mucosa: nomenclature and classification. Rev Stomatol Chir Maxillofac 2010; 111: 208-211.

5- Chung CH, Yang YH, Wang TY, Shieh TY, Warnakulasuriya S

Oral precancerous disorders associated with areca quid chewing, smoking, and alcohol drinking in southern Taiwan.

J Oral Pathol Med. 2005 Sep;34(8):460-6.

6- J Bánóczy, Z Gintner, C Dombi.

Tobacco Use and Oral Leukoplakia.

J Dental Education 2001; 65: 322-327.

7- internet source on the link :

oral cavity cancer

https://www.cancer-environnement.fr/fiches/cancers/cancer-de-la-cavite-oral-oral/

8- Thiéry G1 , Gal M1 , Brau JJ2 , Coulet O1 , Odin G3

BETEL QUID AND ORAL CANCERS: A CASE REPORT OBSERVATION

Med Trop2008; 68: 176-178

9- Brad W. Neville, DDS;Terry A. Day, MD, FACS

Oral Cancer and Precancerous Lesions

CA Cancer J Clin 2002;52:195-215

10- anatomy and histology of the oral mucosa
https://dermatologiebuccale-nice.fr/anatomie-et-histologie-de-la-muqueuse-buccal/histology-of-the-mucosa-buccal

11- Anne-Laure Ejeil, Maddy-Hélène Delattre, Nathan Moreau

The oral mucosa and its pathophysiological alterations

12- Stephen Porter, PhD,a Luiz Alcino Gueiros, PhD,b Jair Carneiro Leão, PhD,b and Stefano Fedele, PhD

Risk factors and etiopathogenesis of potentially premalignant oral epithelial lesions

Oral Surg Oral Med Oral Pathol Oral Radiol 2018;125:603-611

13- Yen-Wen Shen ,Yin-Hwa Shih, Lih-Jyh Fuh, Tzong-Ming Shieh

Oral Submucous Fibrosis: A Review on Biomarkers, Pathogenic Mechanisms, and Treatments

Int. J. Mol. Sci. 2020, *27*(19), 7231

14- Saman Warnakulasuriya, FDS, PhD, DSca

Clinical features and presentation of oral potentially malignant disorders

(Oral Surg Oral Med Oral Pathol Oral Radiol 2018;125:582-590)

15- Antony George, Sreenivasan BS, Sunil S, Soma Susan Varghese, Jubin Thomas, Devi Gopakumar, Varghese Mani.

POTENTIALLY MALIGNANT DISORDE RS OF ORAL CAVITY

Oral & Maxillofacial Pathology Journal ; V ol 2. No 1 ; Jan- Jun 2011. ISSN 0976-1225

16- Lorini, L.; Bescós Atín, C.; Thavaraj, S.; Müller-Richter, U.; Alberola Ferranti, M.; Pamias Romero, J.; Sáez Barba, M.; de Pablo García-Cuenca, A.; Braña García, I.; Bossi, P.; et al.

Overview of Oral Potentially Malignant Disorders: From Risk Factors to Specific Therapies Cancers 2021, 13,
3696.

17- Sonia Gupta and Manveen Kaur **JawandaOral Lichen Planus: An Update on Etiology, Pathogenesis, Clinical Presentation, Diagnosis and** ManagementIndian J Dermatol. 2015 May-Jun; 60(3): 222-229.

18- STELLA LYSITSA, SEEMAN ABI NAJM, TOMMASO LOMBARDI,
JACKY SAMSON **Oral lichen planus: natural history and malignant transformation**
Med Buccale Chir Buccale 2007; 13: 19-29.

19- internet source : **Malignant Potential Lesion of the Buccal Mucosa link:https://opmdcare.com/category/lesion-a-potentiel-malin-de-la-muq ueuse-buccale/?lang= en**

20- https://www.centredentairesjb.com/services/velscope/

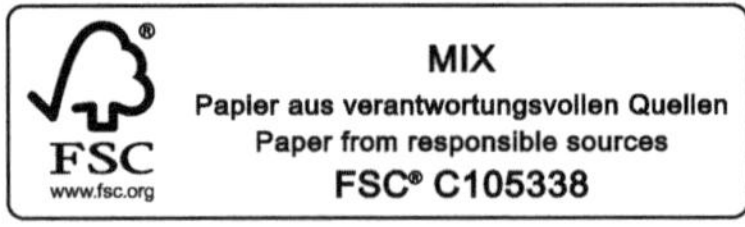

Printed by Books on Demand GmbH, Norderstedt / Germany